Anti Inflammatory Diet: Autoimmune Lunch Recipes

35+ Anti Inflammation Diet Recipes To Fight Autoimmune Disease, Reduce Pain And Restore Health (2nd Edition)

By Kira Novac (ISBN-13: 978-1533313034)

Copyright ©Kira Novac 2016

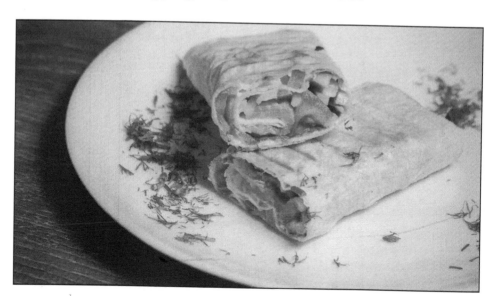

www.amazon.com/author/kira-novac

All information in this book has been carefully researched and checked for factual accuracy. However, the author and publishers make no warranty, expressed or implied, that the information contained herein is appropriate for every individual, situation or purpose, and assume no responsibility for errors or omission. The reader assumes the risk and full responsibility for all actions, and the author will not be held liable for any loss or damage, whether consequential, incidental, and special or otherwise, that may result from the information presented in this publication.

A physician has not written the information in this book. Before making any serious dietary changes, I advise you to consult with your physician first.

Table of contents

Free Complimentary Recipe eBook

Thank you so much for taking an interest in my work!

As a thank you, I would love to offer you a free complimentary recipe eBook to help you achieve vibrant health. It will teach you how to prepare amazingly tasty and healthy gluten-free treats so that you never feel deprived or bored again!

As a special bonus, you will be able to receive all my future books (kindle format) for free or only $0.99.

Download your free recipe eBook here:

http://bit.ly/gluten-free-desserts-book

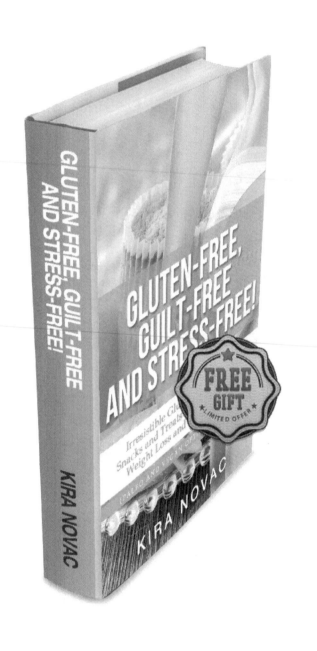

Introduction

Tasty and Healthy Anti-Inflammatory Diet Lunch Recipes

What *is* inflammation? Inflammation is a commonly used term these days, but let's think about what it really means. Inflammation can be healthy and natural, for example if we get a cut and our bodies' healing mechanism produces redness and swelling. This is a normal inflammatory response.

However, the problem comes in when we are dealing with chronic, systemic inflammation. This occurs when our body is suffering from chronic stressors, which could be physical, mental/emotional, or environmental in nature, and are causing long-standing inflammation that affects our bodies' systems. These stressors could be too much work and not enough rest and relaxation, a physical trauma (like an accident or even a childbirth...anything that is hard on the body), a death in the family, OR an environmental factor such as pollutants, toxins, and inflammatory foods.

Some stressors we simply cannot control, unfortunately. But some we can, and food is certainly one of them. Regularly eating a diet high in inflammatory foods such as rancid oils (soy, corn, canola oils, for example), fried foods, refined sugar, baked goods such as cookies, cakes, and pastries, sodas and fruit drinks, and/or commercially raised meats, causes major stress on the body, and this in turn creates inflammation.

In this book, you will find delicious and easy-to-prepare lunch recipes, filled with nutrient dense and anti-inflammatory ingredients. While not noted in each recipe, remember that the quality of your ingredients is of utmost importance. As much as possible, opt for grass-fed meat, organic poultry, wild-caught, fresh fish, and organic produce. This goes a long way in preventing and calming systemic inflammation.

Choose the recipes here that work best for your lifestyle and appeal to your tastes, there are lots to choose from!

Here's to our health!

Anti-inflammatory diet is not a diet really, but a lifestyle. I have included a whole variety of recipes and I divided them into different sections so that it's easier for you to focus on what you and your family prefer.

Shall you have any questions about this book, please email me at:

kira.novac@kiraglutenfreerecipes.com

This book is designed as a simple and practical recipe book. If you wish to learn more about anti-inflammatory diet concepts, check out my book: "Anti-Inflammatory Diet: The Holistic Approach".

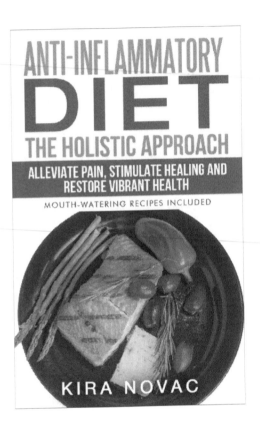

Book Link: http://bit.ly/ai-diet-holistic-approach

Part I

Paleo Recipes

Chard and Spinach Salmon Salad with Pesto

Serves: 4

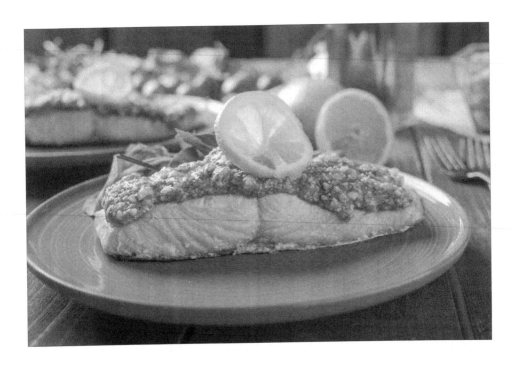

For this recipe, you can use canned or fresh salmon, depending on availability and your timeframe. Salmon is rich in anti-inflammatory omega 3 fatty acids, and chard and spinach are 2 leafy green vegetables packed full of important nutrients like the mineral magnesium, which is essential for rest and relaxation. And top it off, it tastes delicious!

INGREDIENTS:

Pesto:

- 2 cups fresh basil leaves
- 2 garlic cloves
- ¼ cup walnuts or pine nuts
- ½ cup extra virgin olive oil
- salt and pepper to taste

Salad:

- 2 cups spinach (regular or baby)
- 2 cups chard, chopped
- ½ cup cilantro, chopped
- ½ cup parsley, chopped
- ½ beet, shredded
- ½ carrot, shredded
- 1 cup snap peas, de-stemmed
- Juice of 1 fresh lemon
- Salmon (if not using canned):

- 1 lb. salmon (16 oz, preferably wild Alaskan if possible)
- Salt and pepper to taste

INSTRUCTIONS:

1. Using a food processor (or high quality blender), mix together your basil, garlic, walnuts or pine nuts until totally smooth. Then, begin slowly adding olive oil until mixture is smooth. Taste and add salt and pepper accordingly.
2. Next, prepare the salmon (if making fresh). Preheat oven to 400 degrees. In a baking dish, add salmon and top with pesto, adding a bit more salt and pepper. Bake until done, anywhere from 20-45 minutes depending on thickness. Check frequently.
3. Assemble your salad. In a large bowl, add together all salad ingredients, top with lemon juice and toss.
4. Top salad with salmon and serve.

Turkey Lettuce Wrap
Serves: 2

The beauty of a lettuce wrap is that you can wrap up just about anything! Similarly, you can most any hamburger recipe and turn it into a lettuce wrap, making it a far healthier option. Include your favorite veggies, meat/protein options hot sauce or spices and enjoy! This particular wrap uses ground turkey, and is quick, easy and delicious.

INGREDIENTS:

- 1 lb. ground turkey
- 2 cloves garlic, minced
- 1 tbsp. ground flax seeds
- 1 tomato, thinly sliced
- ¼ red onion, finely chopped
- ½ tsp. cayenne (optional)
- ¼ cup basil leaves, finely chopped
- Salt and pepper to taste
- Hot sauce (optional)
- Romaine or butter lettuce leaves for wrapping

INSTRUCTIONS:

1. In a bowl, thoroughly mix together your ground turkey, flax seeds, garlic, onion, cayenne, basil, salt and pepper. Use a fork or even your hands to mix well.

2. Now, form patties into your desired size and cook in a frying pan, about 5 minutes on each side or until cooked through.

3. On a plate (or Tupperware if packing), arrange lettuce leaves topped with a turkey burger, tomato slices, and hot sauce (if using). Wrap up and enjoy!

Steak and Peach Salad
Serves: 2-4

Who wouldn't look forward to steak for lunch? This unique salad offers not only a wonderful array of flavors, but also the myriad of nutrient benefits that come from grass-fed steak, like a high dose of healthy omega 3 fatty acids. Use peaches if available, or your favorite seasonal fruit (berries could be delicious too, and are rich in antioxidants). Or add both!

INGREDIENTS:

- ¼ cup flax or olive oil
- 2 tbsp. almond butter
- 4 cups mixed salad greens of your choice
- 1-2 cups thinly sliced and cooked steak (depending how many people you are feeding)
- 1 cup sliced peaches (or other seasonal fruit)
- 1 tomato, sliced
- ¼ cup thinly sliced red onion
- 1 large avocado, peeled and thinly sliced
- 2 tbsp. balsamic vinegar
- 2 tbsp. olive oil

- 1 ½ tsp. grade b or c maple syrup

INSTRUCTIONS:

1. First, assemble your dressing. Vigorously mix or whisk together olive oil, almond butter, balsamic vinegar and maple syrup. Set aside.
2. In a large salad bowl, place your greens. Top with steak, onions, tomato, peaches and avocado. Add dressing, mix together and serve.

Paleo Sweet Potato Boat
Serves: 2

This tasty vegetable is packed with important nutrients such as vitamins A and C, manganese and copper. It is more nutrient dense than a potato, and a much healthier source of carbohydrate than rice or bread. This dish is one of my favorites, satisfying and rich in its flavor profile.

INGREDIENTS:

- 2 large sweet potatoes
- 1 onion, chopped
- 16 oz. mushrooms (your choice, crimini work well), quartered
- 3 garlic cloves, minced
- 8-12 oz. cooked and shredded chicken
- 1 tsp. dried thyme
- 2-3 cups mixed salad greens of your choice
- Olive oil and balsamic vinegar for dressing (or fresh lemon juice)
- Salt and pepper to taste

INSTRUCTIONS:

1. First, bake your sweet potato by poking holes in it with a fork and placing it in the oven for about 45 minutes or until fork-soft. Remove and allow to cool enough to handle.

2. Next, slice the potato in half (lengthwise), and spoon out most of the meat, leaving enough layering the skin so that it stays intact. Chop or mash the meat of the potato.

3. Heat a sauté pan on medium heat and add your sweet potato meat, onion, garlic, mushrooms, chicken, thyme, salt and pepper. Stir constantly until vegetables are cooked.

4. Now, remove from sauté pan and place into a large bowl, mixing in salad greens. Scoop this mixture back into your potato skins (boats) and top with a bit of olive oil and balsamic vinegar or lemon juice.

Paleo Lunchbox Medley
Serves: 1

Channel your inner child here as if you're packing a fun array of lunchbox foods! You can get creative, but here you have an even and healthy mix of your 3 macronutrients: protein, fat and carbohydrates. This can be a great on the go option, and you can prepare it quickly for the whole family.

INGREDIENTS:

- 2 eggs, hardboiled
- 1 tomato, sliced
- ½ avocado, sliced
- ½ cucumber, sliced
- ½ apple, sliced
- ½ banana, sliced
- 1 serving dark chocolate (70% or higher)
- 1 tsp. ground cinnamon
- Salt and pepper

INSTRUCTIONS:

1. Not much to explain here, simply assemble all of your ingredients in a Tupperware, top eggs, cucumber, tomato and avocado with a touch of salt and pepper and sprinkle cinnamon on your chopped fruit (optional).
2. Enjoy!

Casserole
Serves: 5

This is a wonderful option for both breakfast and lunch (or dinner, for that matter), and the best part is that it keeps well in the fridge or freezer. You can make it ahead of time and grab it on the go, or prepare and eat fresh. It offers a healthy serving of protein and good fat to keep you satiated throughout the day and help ward off sugar cravings.

INGREDIENTS:

- 2 tbsp. coconut oil, ghee or butter, melted
- 1 sweet potato or yam, washed and diced
- 1 ½ lbs. breakfast sausage or ground meat of your choice
- ½ onion, finely chopped
- 2 cloves garlic, minced
- 2 cups spinach, chard or kale, chopped
- 10 eggs, whisked
- ¾ tsp. salt

INSTRUCTIONS:

1. First, preheat your oven to 400 degrees.
2. Mix your diced sweet potatoes or yams with the melted oil (or other fat of choice), along with salt.
3. In a greased 9 x 12 baking dish, place your sweet potato mixture and bake for about 20 minutes. Remove once to stir.
4. Now (or while your sweet potatoes cook), heat your breakfast sausage or other ground meat in a sauté pan over medium-high heat with chopped onion. Stir constantly until the meat is completely cooked.
5. Remove the sweet potatoes from the oven and add in meat, eggs, spinach (or other greens), garlic powder, salt and pepper and mix well.
6. Cook in the oven for another 25 minutes, or until eggs or cooked through. Enjoy!

Delicious Tuna Burger
Serves: 1-2

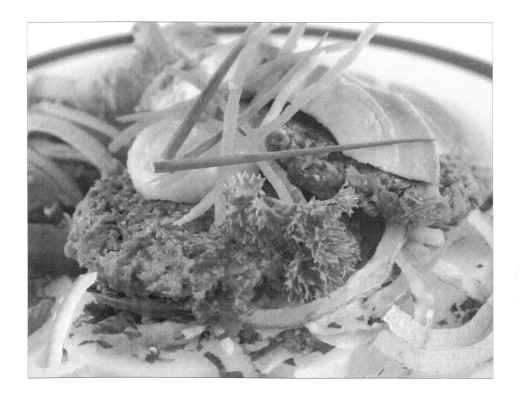

This paleo lunch option is quick, easy and inexpensive. They can also be made ahead of time. Tuna (in water) is a great source of omega 3 fatty acids, and these use coconut flour instead of wheat that contains gluten, which is very inflammatory for some people. You can get creative about toppings for these burgers, and definitely serve with a side salad, as including dark, leafy greens as much as possible is key for fighting inflammation.

INGREDIENTS:

- 1 can tuna, drained
- 1 small onion, finely diced
- 1 small red chili (optional if you like spice), chopped finely
- 2 garlic cloves, minced
- 1 egg
- 2 tbsp. tomato paste
- 1 tbsp. coconut flour
- Lettuce, avocado, tomato can be used for toppings
- Salt and pepper to taste

INSTRUCTIONS:

1. Preheat your oven to 350 degrees.
2. In a mixing bowl, mix together tuna, onion, chili (if using), garlic, egg, tomato paste and coconut flour. Mix thoroughly until you have a thick consistency.
3. Next, form your tuna mixture into patties of your desired size. Place them onto a greased baking sheet.
4. Bake in the oven for 10 minutes (or less, check regularly), until they are done.

5. Serve (or pack for lunch) with toppings of choice, and of course a salad on the side.

Part II

Vegetarian Recipes

Chickpea and Spinach Medley
Serves: 4

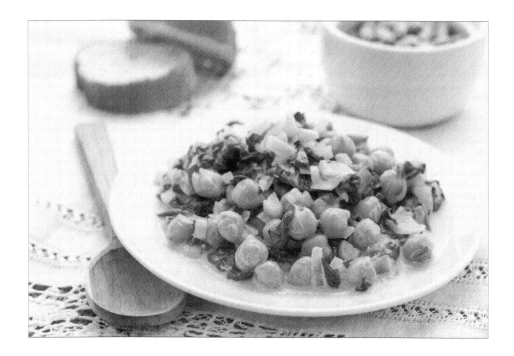

Garbanzo beans (chickpeas) are a great vegetarian source of protein, and are high in minerals and vitamins molybdenum, manganese, folate, iron and zinc. They are also an excellent source of fiber, which is important in any anti-inflammatory diet in order to achieve and maintain healthy digestion.

INGREDIENTS:

- 1 lb. spinach
- 1 ½ tbsp. extra virgin olive oil
- 1 onion, finely chopped
- 3 garlic cloves, minced
- 1 12 oz. can chickpeas, washed and drained
- 1 tsp. dried thyme
- 1 tsp. oregano
- 1 tsp. cumin
- 1 tsp. sea salt
- ¼ cup raisins
- ¼ cup vegetable broth (organic store-bought or homemade)

INSTRUCTIONS:

1. Rinse and dry your spinach, placing it, one handful at a time to a pot on medium heat, stirring/tossing constantly until all spinach is just wilted. Now, remove from heat and chop.

2. In a sauté pan on medium heat, add your olive oil until heated. Next, add in onion and garlic, stirring until onion is

translucent and garlic is browned, being careful not to burn.

3. Next, add in garbanzo beans, thyme, oregano, paprika, cumin and salt and mash some of your chickpeas with either the back of a fork or a potato masher (leave some whole). Cook everything while stirring constantly for about 5 minutes.

4. Lastly, add in raising, broth and spinach, stirring until everything is heated together. Top with remaining olive oil and serve.

Black Bean-Zucchini Stir-Fry
Serves: 4

This comforting and tasty anti-inflammatory recipe is quick to prepare and packed with nutrients. Black beans are also a great source of fiber and protein, and brown rice holds more nutrient value than its white-rice counterpart. Zucchini is an excellent source of copper and vitamin C, both important for cooling inflammation and immune health.

INGREDIENTS:

- 1 tbsp. extra virgin olive oil
- 1 2 cups zucchini squash, sliced
- 1 cup bell pepper, diced
- 1 can black beans, drained and rinsed
- 1 can diced tomatoes
- ¾ cup water
- 1 cup brown rice

INSTRUCTIONS:

1. First, cook your rice in a pot over the stove. Place 1 ½ cups water and rice in the pot, covered. Bring everything to a boil, then immediately lower to a simmer and allow to cook until rice is done, around 20 minutes. You can even add a spoonful of coconut oil or butter and a pinch of salt to give it some extra flavor and texture.

2. Next, heat olive oil in a sauté pan over medium heat, adding zucchini and bell pepper. Cook for about 5 minutes, constantly stirring.

3. Add your black beans, tomatoes and water, and cook all together until heated. Add your rice to the mixture once it is fully cooked, and continue heating for another 5 minutes or so.

4. Serve and enjoy!

Delicious Cheesy Tomatoes
Serves: 2

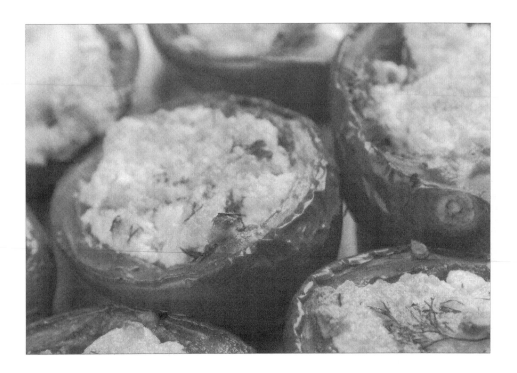

This recipe is wonderful for a chilly day when you're craving comfort food like lasagna. Instead, opt for this much healthier alternative, while still indulging in the comfort and tastiness of your winter day favorites. Tomatoes are rich in anti-inflammatory antioxidants, and olive oil is a healthy source of dietary fat. This recipe is also usually a kid-favorite, so the entire family can enjoy! Serve with a green side salad.

INGREDIENTS:

- 4 tomatoes, cut in half
- ¼ grated fresh parmesan cheese
- 1 ½ tsp. oregano
- 1 tsp. basil (fresh or dried)
- ½ tsp. sea salt
- Black pepper to taste
- 4 tbsp. extra virgin olive oil

INSTRUCTIONS:

1. Begin by preheating your oven to 450 degrees.
2. On a baking sheet, place your halved tomatoes face up, and top with parmesan cheese, oregano, basil, salt and pepper. Then, drizzle each tomato with olive oil.
3. Bake for 10-15 minutes, or until tomatoes are soft, and serve with a salad.

Healthy Mozzarella Tomato Sandwich
Serves: 1

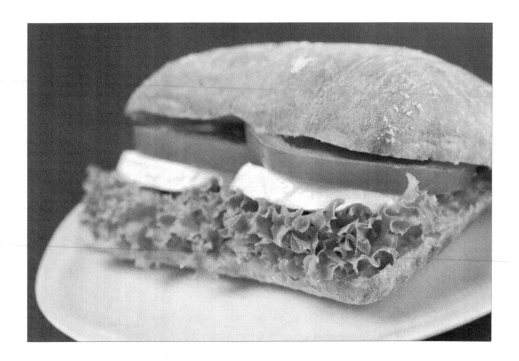

While bread is not my first choice in an anti-inflammatory diet, if eaten only occasionally, it shouldn't be a problem (assuming you don't have a gluten sensitivity or allergy). For this recipe, opt for a multi-grain loaf, OR a gluten free option. My favorite part of this sandwich is that it incorporates the fresh herbs parsley and cilantro, which are great for detoxification and packed full of essential nutrients.

INGREDIENTS:

- 2 tbsp. Dijon mustard (or your favorite kind)
- ½ cup sun-dried tomatoes in oil, drained (save about 1 tbsp. of oil)
- 2 slices multi-grain or gluten free bread
- Lettuce leaves
- 4 oz. fresh mozzarella cheese, thinly sliced
- ¼ cup fresh parsley
- ¼ cup fresh cilantro
- Salt and pepper to taste

INSTRUCTIONS:

1. First, lightly toast your bread slices.
2. In a bowl, vigorously stir or whisk together your olive oil and mustard until it thickens. Use this to spread onto your two slices of bread.
3. Arrange your sandwich with lettuce, cheese, tomatoes, cilantro and parsley. Top with salt and pepper. Serve.

Kale Burrito Bowl
Serves: 4-5

Many of us know by now that Kale is a super-food, but why? Kale offers some amazing cholesterol lowering benefits, and is packed full of nutrients and fiber. It is loaded with 45 different flavonoids, all key for fighting inflammation and preventing illness. Kale provides over 1000% of the RDA for vitamin D, along with high levels of vitamins A and C. This recipe is not only delicious, but a super healthy option for vegetarians and non-vegetarians alike!

INGREDIENTS:

Rice:

- 1 cup brown or jasmine rice
- 2 cups water

Kale:

- 1 bunch of kale (your choice of which type), chopped
- ½ cup fresh lemon juice

- 2 tbsp. olive or avocado oil
- ½ jalapeno pepper, diced
- ½ tsp. cumin
- Salt and pepper to taste

Avocado Salsa:

- 1 avocado, sliced
- 2 tomatoes, finely chopped
- 1 jalapeno pepper, diced
- ½ cup cilantro leaves, finely chopped
- ½ red onion, finely chopped
- Juice of 1 lemon

Black Beans:

- 2 cans black beans rinsed and drained, OR 2 cups beans soaked and cooked
- ½ onion, finely chopped
- 3 garlic cloves, minced
- ½ tsp. chili powder

INSTRUCTIONS:

1. First, cook your rice. Place rice and water in a saucepan, adding a pinch of salt. Bring to a boil, then lower to a simmer and cover until rice is done, about 30 minutes.

2. While rice is cooking, prepare kale salad by whisking together lemon juice, olive oil, jalapeno pepper, salt and cumin. Whisk all together, and pour over your chopped kale and massage dressing into kale leaves until they are soft, about 2-3 minutes.

3. Next, mix together all avocado salsa ingredients in a mixing bowl.

4. Moving onto the beans, heat 1 tbsp. olive oil in a sauté pan, adding your onions and garlic and cooking for 3 minutes, stirring constantly. Next, add your beans and chili powder.

5. Stir bean mixture until heated.

6. Time to serve! In bowls, serve equal amounts of rice, beans and kale salad, topped with avocado salsa. Enjoy!

Veggie Wrap
Serves: 1

The beauty of the wrap is that you can be super creative, adding your favorite ingredients and/or whatever you have on hand. This version has hummus, which is not only tasty but provides protein, along with avocado for an excellent healthy fat, along with various veggies, which up the nutrient value of this lunch dish.

INGREDIENTS:

- 1 whole wheat or sprouted grain wrap (or gluten free)
- 2-3 tbsp. organic hummus (your favorite kind)
- ½ cucumber, sliced
- ¼ carrot, grated
- 2 tbsp. olives
- ½ avocado, sliced
- 1 tbsp. olive oil
- Juice from ½ fresh lemon
- 1 oz. feta cheese (optional)
- Salt and pepper to taste

INSTRUCTIONS:

These are very easy to assemble, so prep time is kept at a minimal. Simply spread humus onto your wrap of choice, and top with all remaining veggies, avocado, cheese, lemon juice and olive oil. Add salt and pepper to taste, wrap up and enjoy!

Bean Burrito
Serves: 1

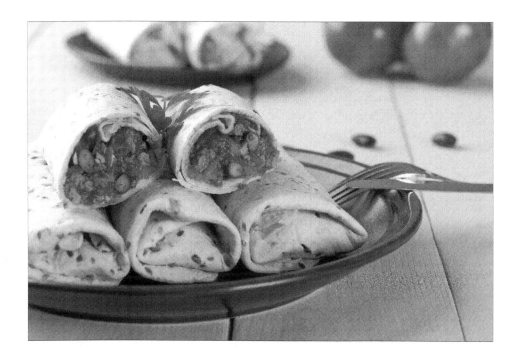

This is another quick and easy vegetarian option, and can be made with several variations. You could use red or pinto beans, although this recipe calls for black beans, which are not only high in fiber but offer copper, folate, vitamin B1 and magnesium. Be sure to buy BPA free cans, as this toxic found in the lining of many canned foods can be dangerous to your health.

INGREDIENTS:

- Whole wheat or sprouted grain tortilla (or make 2 smaller burritos using corn tortillas)
- ½ cup black beans, rinsed and drained if from a can, or homemade
- 1 cup shredded lettuce
- ½ avocado, sliced
- 1-2 oz. cheddar cheese, shredded
- Salsa (organic, store-bought or homemade)

INSTRUCTIONS:

Similarly to the previous recipe, this takes only minutes to prepare. Lay out your tortilla and arrange all toppings. Wrap up and enjoy! Other great additions could be fresh, diced onion, diced tomato, cilantro and hot sauce.

Part III

Vegan Recipes

Taco Salad
Serves: 2

This unique recipe isn't only vegan, it's also raw. In any diet (vegan or not), it is important to get a mix of both cooked and raw vegetables, as both offer different nutrient value. This delicious salad uses sunflower seeds, which are particularly high in vitamin E and copper, and offer protein. You are also getting a great dose of vitamins and minerals from all of the veggies, and good fats from the avocado.

INGREDIENTS:

Sunflower "Meat":

- ½ cup sunflower seeds, soaked for at least 2 hours (up to 8, you can also use walnuts here as an alternative)
- 1 tsp. chili powder
- 1 tsp. cumin
- ½ tsp. cayenne pepper
- Salt to taste

Cashew Cream:

- 1 cup cashew nuts, soaked for at least 2 hours (up to 8)
- 1-2 cups water (depending on how thick you want it)
- Juice of 1 fresh lemon
- Salt to taste

Guacamole:

- 1 avocado
- 1/3 cup onion, chopped
- 1 tomato, chopped
- 1 tsp cumin
- Juice of 1 fresh lemon
- Salt to taste

Salad:

- 4 cups mixed greens of choice
- Salsa (organic, store-bought or homemade)

INSTRUCTIONS:

1. Begin by preparing your "meat." Using a food processor if you have one, or simply by hand, chop you seeds (or walnuts) together with the spices.

2. Now for the cashew sauce. Rinse and drain the cashews after they've soaked, and place them in a food processor with ½ cup water to start. Add 2 tbsp. lemon juice, and continue adding water as needed depending on thickness. It should be very smooth.

3. Assemble the guacamole by mixing together all ingredients in a bowl. Mash the avocado with a fork (or your hand), and mix together well with everything else. Add salt to taste.

4. Lastly, arrange your salad. In your serving bowls, add greens and top with guacamole. Next, add salsa and taco "meat" (divided evenly between each salad). On top, place the raw chopped onion and tomato, and drizzle lemon juice on top if you'd like.

Vegan Chili
Serves: 4

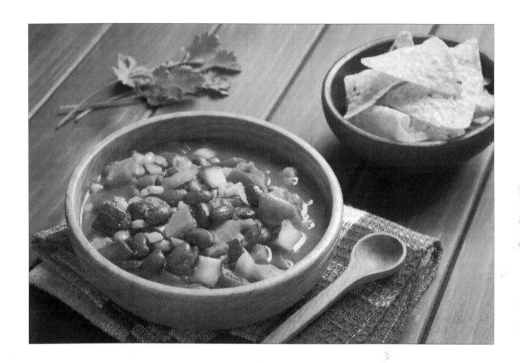

This is a wonderful option on a cold day, or simply if you want a heartier lunch option. This delicious chili recipe has a unique and rich flavor profile, and two types of beans, which are essential for fiber and protein, particularly if following a vegan diet. Like most soups and chilies, you can easily freeze this for lunches and dinners throughout the week.

INGREDIENTS:

- 2 tbsp. extra virgin olive oil
- 2 cups diced red onion
- 3 cloves garlic, minced
- 1-2 jalapeno peppers, diced (optional)
- 1 green bell pepper, finely chopped
- 1 cup celery, finely chopped
- 1 28 oz. can diced tomatoes
- 1 cup vegetable broth (store bought or homemade)
- 6 tbsp. tomato paste
- 1 can kidney beans
- 1 can pinto beans
- 2 tsp. cumin
- 2 tbsp. chili powder
- 1 tsp. oregano
- ½ tsp. cayenne pepper (optional)
- Salt and pepper to taste

Toppings:

Choose your favorite chili toppings, such as vegan sour cream or fresh cilantro.

INSTRUCTIONS:

1. In a large soup pot, heat your olive oil on medium heat. Add onion and garlic, stirring until onion is soft, then add a bit of salt.

2. Next, add jalapenos (if using), bell pepper and celery, stirring together for about 5 minutes.

3. Next, add diced tomatoes, veggie broth, and tomato paste, stirring until thoroughly combined. Increase heat to medium-high.

4. Add pinto and kidney beans along with all other spices (chili, cumin, oregano, cayenne and salt). Simmer until your chili becomes thick, for roughly 15 minutes.

5. Serve with toppings of your choice.

Black Bean Quinoa Bowl
Serves: 4

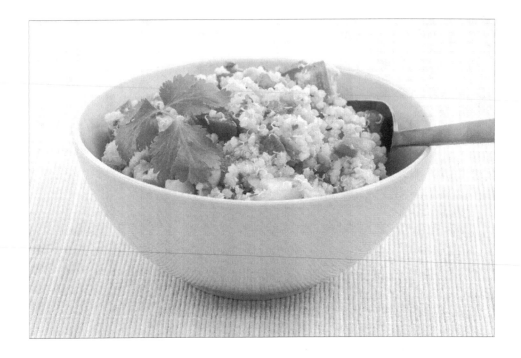

Not only is quinoa a great protein source for vegans, but it also has been found to contain two important antioxidants, quercetin and kaemferol, in high amounts. Contrary to popular belief, quinoa is actually a seed instead of a grain, and is high in manganese, copper, phosphorus and magnesium. This vegan bowl is a delicious lunch time treat.

INGREDIENTS:

Salad:

- 3 cups cooked quinoa (will be about 1 cup raw)
- 1 can black beans, drained and rinsed
- 1 cup cilantro, chopped
- 1 roasted yam or sweet potato
- 1 red onion, thinly sliced
- Salt and pepper to taste
- 1 avocado, sliced
- Vegan or raw crackers of your choice

Dressing:

- Juice of 1 fresh lime
- 2 tbsp. extra virgin olive oil
- 1 garlic clove, minced
- 1 tsp. cumin
- 1-2 tsp. grade b maple syrup
- Salt and pepper to taste

INSTRUCTIONS:

1. If starting with uncooked quinoa, begin by placing it into a pot with 1.5 cups of water, bringing it to a boil, and then simmering with the lid on until done, about 15-20 minutes. Place in the fridge while you prepare the rest of the meal.

2. While quinoa is cooking, prepare your dressing. Whisk together all ingredients or shake in a jar.

3. Remove quinoa and put in a big mixing bowl. Add black beans, sweet potato (or yam), cilantro and onion. Mix everything together.

4. Add dressing, salt and pepper to taste and toss the salad.

5. Serve with sliced avocado and crackers.

Avocado Chickpea Salad
Serves: 2

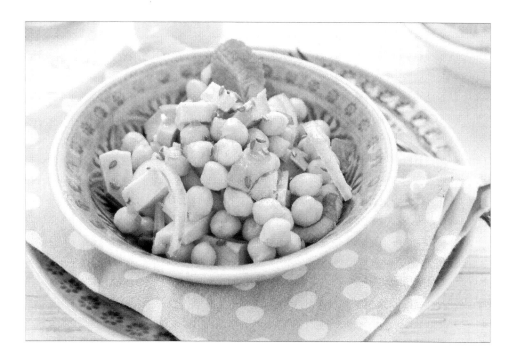

This is a great option for a protein-rich, light lunch. You might consider serving it alongside a roasted sweet potato for a heartier meal, or as is for something on the lighter side. Garbanzo beans are high in fiber, which is essential for healthy digestion, and avocadoes are rich in good fats, which are important for cell maintenance and function, not to mention weight management.

INGREDIENTS:

- 1 can chickpeas, rinsed and drained
- 1 large or 2 small avocadoes, cubed
- ½ cup fresh cilantro leaves, chopped
- ½ red onion, thinly sliced
- juice of 1 fresh lemon
- 2 tbsp. extra virgin olive oil
- salt and pepper to taste

INSTRUCTIONS:

Simply place all ingredients into a big salad bowl and toss together. Top with lemon juice, olive oil, salt and pepper and serve.

Ultimate Vegan Bowl
Serves: 2

This is definitely a heartier lunch option and packed with a huge variety of important macro and micro nutrients, not to mention tastes. Red cabbage offers high amounts of vitamin K, essential to bone health, and vitamin C, essential to immune health. Sweet potatoes are also high in vitamin C and a healthy carbohydrate option, *and* this dish is full of protein.

INGREDIENTS:

- 1 sweet potato, washed and cubed
- 1 can black beans, rinsed and drained (or prepared from scratch)
- 1 cup brown rice or whole grain of choice
- 1 carrot, shredded
- 1 beet, shredded
- ¼ purple cabbage, shredded
- 2 cups kale or other dark leafy green of choice (spinach, Swiss chard, etc)
- juice of 1 fresh lemon
- 1 avocado, sliced

- organic hummus of your choice
- 1 tbsp. coconut oil
- salt and pepper to taste

INSTRUCTIONS:

1. Begin by roasting your sweet potato. Preheat oven to 400 degrees, and place sweet potato cubes in a baking dish tossed evenly with coconut oil and salt and pepper to taste. Bake until sweet potato is tender, about 30 minutes.

2. Next, prepare your grain according to which you have chosen. Typically, this will be about double the amount of water (for example, 1 cup of rice to 2 cups of water), bringing everything to a boil and them lowering to a simmer, covered until cooked.

3. Now, arrange everything together on serving plates. The plate should consist of roasted sweet potato, chickpeas, rice/other grain divided into 2 portions, carrot, cabbage, greens, heaping spoonful of hummus and half an avocado for each. Drizzle with lemon juice and a bit more salt/pepper to taste if desired.

Ultimate Vegan Sandwich
Serves: 1

I've described the last two recipes as 'ultimate' because really it doesn't get much better! This unique and hearty sandwich offers the benefit of fresh basil, which is high in vitamin K and has cell protective flavanoids. This lunch option is high in healthy vegan protein, and will leave you feeling satisfied.

INGREDIENTS:

Pesto:

- 1 cup fresh basil
- ½ cup walnuts (raw if possible)
- 2 garlic cloves
- ¼ extra virgin olive oil
- juice of 1 fresh lemon
- 2 tbsp. purified water
- sea salt and pepper to taste

Sandwich:

- 2 slices multi-grain or sprouted-grain bread (or gluten free, if sensitive)
- 2 tbsp. organic hummus
- 2 tbsp. pesto
- ½ tomato, sliced
- ½ avocado, sliced
- lettuce or spinach

INSTRUCTIONS:

1. Toast your bread slices (optional, but tasty).
2. Begin with preparing the pesto. In a food processor, add all ingredients except the olive oil. As you begin mixing everything together/processing, slowly add your olive oil, little by little, until you have the desired consistency of your pesto.
3. Next, arrange the sandwich. Spread hummus and pesto on your bread slices, and layer with avocado, tomato, and lettuce or spinach.

Part IV

Soup Recipes

Cooling Gazpacho Soup
Serves: 8

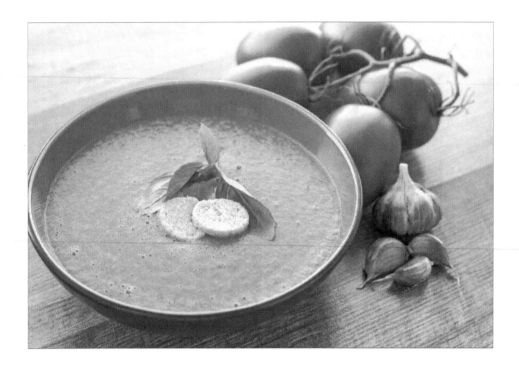

Gazpacho soup is the perfect option on a hot summer day, or if you're wanting a lighter soup option. This recipe offers the rich nutrient content of tomatoes, primarily the antioxidant lycopene, which studies show to be strongly tied to bone health. Serve this with a green salad and enjoy its' cooling properties!

INGREDIENTS:

- 4 large tomatoes, peeled and chopped
- 2 medium sized cucumbers, peeled and chopped
- 1 cup red bell pepper, finely chopped
- 1 large yellow onion, finely chopped
- 3 cups tomato juice (canned or better yet simply blend tomatoes in a blender)
- 2 tbsp. fresh thyme leaves
- ½ cup red wine vinegar
- 3 cloves garlic, peeled and minced
- 2 tbsp. canned tomato paste
- Juice of 1 lemon
- Salt and pepper to taste
- Cayenne pepper to taste (optional)

INSTRUCTIONS:

1. First, set aside 3 tbsp. each of bell pepper, tomato, onion and cucumber.
2. Next, puree all remaining ingredients in a blender until completely smooth and creamy. Add more lemon juice, salt, pepper and cayenne if desired.

3. Place soup in a bowl and refrigerate for a minimum of 2 hours, but preferably overnight. If soup thickens too much, you can always mix in a bit of water.

4. That's it! Serve in bowls and garnish with the ingredients you initially set aside.

Comforting Carrot Ginger Soup
Serves 4

Ginger root has a myriad of anti-inflammatory properties. In fact, if you are experiencing digestive upset, simply chop and boil a chunk of ginger to make a tea! This soup is perfect for not only its' nutrient content, but its unique blend of flavors. Serve with a side salad or coconut muffins (see dessert recipes).

INGREDIENTS:

- 12 carrots sliced
- 1/2 yellow onion dices
- 3 tablespoons minced ginger
- 3 cups vegetable broth
- 2 tablespoon
- olive oil
- salt to taste

INSTRUCTIONS:

1. Sauté onion and ginger with olive oil on medium heat in a large pan until onions appear translucent.

2. Add carrots, combining and stirring with sautéed onion and ginger for 1 minute. Add vegetable broth, cover, bring to a boil and let simmer for about 15 minutes or until carrots are soft.

3. When finished, put ingredients through blender. I recommend letting the mixture cool first before blending. This recipe is great with the coconut flour muffins mentioned above, or your favorite multi-grain or gluten free bread.

Butternut Squash Soup
Serves: 4

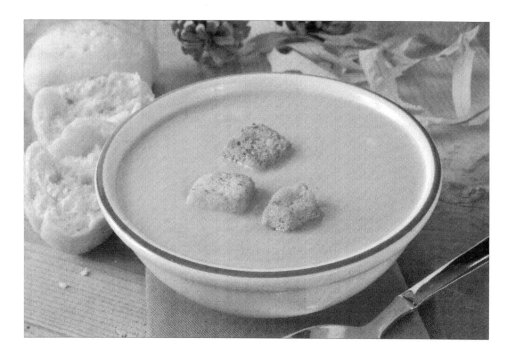

This is absolutely a fall favorite. Sweet butternut squash is so tasty on its own, you definitely don't need to add any sweetener, although this dish almost tastes like dessert! Butternut squash is full of cancer fighting antioxidants and vitamin C, and coconut is a medium chain fatty acid that actually aids in weight loss. Serve with a side salad.

INGREDIENTS:

- 1 medium-large butternut squash, halved and de-seeded
- 1 onion, chopped
- 2-3 cups veggie or chicken broth (store bought or homemade)
- 1 tbsp. organic butter, coconut oil or ghee
- ¼ cup coconut milk
- 1 tsp cinnamon
- 1 tsp nutmeg
- ½ tsp cumin
- salt and pepper to taste

INSTRUCTIONS:

1. First, preheat your oven to 400 degrees and place both halves of the squash in the oven. Roast until fork-tender, and remove to let cool.
2. In a soup pot, add your cooking fat of choice (butter, coconut oil, or ghee), and sauté on medium-high heat with onion. Stir constantly until onion is translucent.
3. Once the squash is done, remove from the skin with a spoon and place into the soup pot with the onion.

4. Add cinnamon, nutmeg, cumin, coconut milk, broth and salt and pepper to taste. Using an immersion blender (or regular if needed), blend all ingredients together.

5. When everything is thoroughly blender, heat and allow to cook for another 10 minutes, adding more spices accordingly if desired. Serve!

Tomato Basil Soup
Serves: 5-6

This soup brings me back to childhood, and is delicious served with your favorite multi-grain, sprouted-grain or gluten free bread, along with a green salad. It is also quick and easy to prepare, and will freeze well for later use. Try this soup as-is, or add chicken for extra protein and a heavier lunch. Remember, this soup is high in good fats, so is pretty satiating by itself.

INGREDIENTS:

- 2 cups tomato juice
- 2 cups vegetable or chicken broth (store-bought or homemade)
- 1 28 oz. can crushed tomatoes
- ½ cup fresh basil leaves
- 1 cup coconut milk
- 3 tbsp. organic butter
- salt and pepper to taste

INSTRUCTIONS:

1. This soup is pretty easy to prepare. Combine all ingredients in a soup pot except for the coconut milk and butter. Blend with an immersion blender (or regular if you don't have an immersion).

2. Once all ingredients are blended, simmer for 30 minutes.

3. Lastly, add your butter and coconut milk and stir, letting everything cook for another few minutes. Serve!

Pumpkin Soup
Serves: 4-5

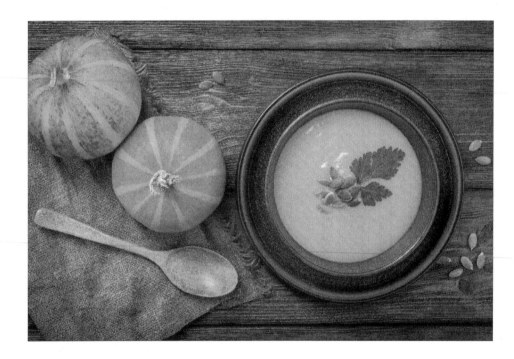

While similar to butternut squash soup in some aspects, this is another great, hearty and healthy soup option. Use your favorite kind of pumpkin, depending on taste preference and what is available locally. And, don't forget to roast the seeds while you're at it, as these are very high in zinc, which is essential for immune support. The meat of the pumpkin is full of important antioxidants, so you can enjoy this soup while knowing you're giving your body the nutrients it needs. Serve with a green salad.

INGREDIENTS:

- 1 pumpkin
- 2 white onions, finely chopped
- 4 garlic cloves, minced
- 2 tbsp. thyme
- 4 cups veggie or chicken broth
- 2 tbsp. extra virgin olive oil

INSTRUCTIONS:

1. Preheat your oven to 400 degrees. With a good quality knife (and carefully!) cut your pumpkin in half and remove the seeds. Place face down on a baking dish or tray and place in the oven, roasting until fork-tender (up to an hour, depending on the size of the pumpkin).

2. In a large soup pot, add olive oil and heat on medium heat, cooking onion and garlic until soft.

3. Once pumpkin is cooked and has cooled enough to handle, scoop out the flesh and add to the soup pot.

4. Now, add in your stock and thyme. Using an immersion (or regular) blender, blend soup until smooth. Enjoy!

Root Vegetable Soup
Serves: 4

Root vegetables are generally going to be more filling, so they make a great soup option. They are also packed with nutrients, and in this soup make a wonderful option for a chilly day. This soup freezes well, so feel free to double the recipe and use it for leftovers. A great variation could be adding 3 or 4 slices of uncured bacon (believe it or not, good quality bacon can be a healthy choice once in a while).

INGREDIENTS:

- 2 tbsp. organic butter, coconut or extra virgin olive oil
- 1 large onion, chopped
- 3 parsnips
- 6 carrots
- 2 beets
- 1-quart veggie, chicken or beef broth
- 2 quarts filtered water
- salt and pepper to taste
- 1 tsp. thyme
- 1 tsp. rosemary

INSTRUCTIONS:

1. In a large soup pot, add your fat of choice (oils mentioned above), and add your onion on medium heat. Stir until onion is soft, about 5-7 minutes.

2. Now, wash all of your root veggies (beet, carrot and parsnips), and cut into medium-sized pieces (depending on how big you want them).

3. When onions are soft, add thyme and rosemary, stirring for 2 minutes with onion.

4. Next, add your chopped root vegetables and mix everything together, allowing to cook for 10 minutes.

5. Add broth and water to the pot and bring to a boil, then reduce to a simmer and cover.

6. Allow to cook until vegetables are tender, about 1 1/2 -2 hours. Add salt and pepper to taste, adjusting other spices if needed, and serve.

Kale Bean Stew
Serves: 4

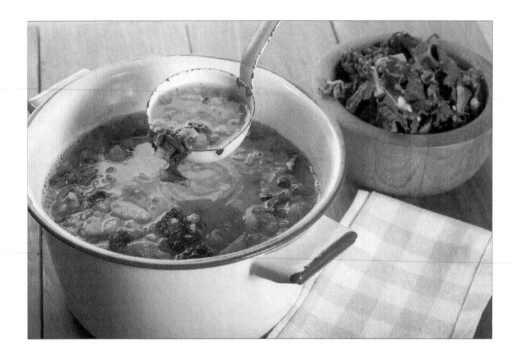

This soup option offers more protein than the last several options, and the myriad of benefits from the super-food, kale. Kale is very high in magnesium, a mineral essential for allowing all of the cells of our body to relax. Navy beans are incredibly rich in fiber, copper and folate.

INGREDIENTS:

- 1 tbsp. extra virgin olive oil
- 4 garlic cloves, minced
- ½ onion, finely chopped
- 2 cups kale, stems removed and chopped
- 2 carrots, washed and chopped
- 2 cups vegetable or chicken broth
- 1 15 oz. cup navy beans, rinsed and drained
- 1 16 oz. can diced tomatoes
- 1 tbsp. thyme
- 1 tbsp. oregano
- salt and pepper to taste

INSTRUCTIONS:

1. First, heat your olive oil in a large soup pot over medium heat. Add garlic and onion, cooking until soft.
2. Add your chopped kale to the pot with a splash of water (or if kale leaves are wet, this is sufficient water). Stir until kale softens and appears wilted, about 12 minutes.
3. Add ¾ of your broth and ¾ of the navy beans. Also add carrots, tomatoes, thyme, oregano, salt and pepper. Mix

everything together and bring to a boil, then lower to a simmer and cook for 10 minutes.

4.   In a blender, mix together the rest of your broth and beans until consistency is smooth. Add this mixture to the soup pot and stir.

5.   Continue to simmer for 10-15 minutes, and serve!

Part V:

Under 10-min Lunch Recipes

Smoked Salmon Wraps
Serves: 2

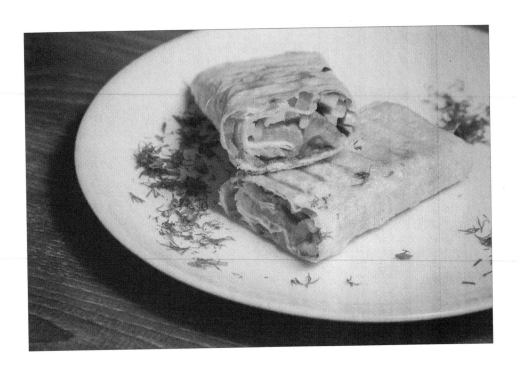

While salmon has a myriad of health benefits (particularly Alaskan King), smoked fish often has added preservatives for shelf life. Be sure to look for a nitrite/nitrate free option, which can be found at your local health food store (Whole Foods, for example). These wraps are quick, easy and delicious and provide healthy, anti-inflammatory fats from both salmon and avocado. You can make the mayonnaise ahead of time, so these can be put together in just a few minutes!

INGREDIENTS:

- 2 wraps of your choice (multigrain, sprouted grain, or gluten free)
- 200 grams of smoked salmon (lox)
- 1 avocado, mashed
- 1 tbsp. homemade paleo mayo (see recipe below)
- 2 tbsp. fresh, chopped dill
- 2 tbsp. mustard
- 1 large carrot, washed and shredded
- 6 lettuce leaves
- Juice of 1 fresh lemon
- Salt and pepper to taste

INSTRUCTIONS:

1. In a mixing bowl, mix together your sliced avocado, dill, homemade mayonnaise, mustard and lemon juice.
2. Lay out your wraps and top with a generous helping of the avocado mixture, spreading evenly. Top with smoked salmon, carrot, and then lettuce.
3. Roll-up, cut in half and pack for lunch!

Paleo Mayonnaise

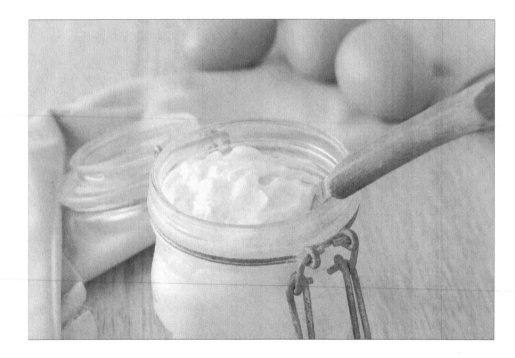

Unlike a store-bought mayonnaise, this option is whole-food based, nutrient dense, and much tastier! It won't keep in the fridge as long as the store-bought version (because it doesn't contain chemical preservatives), so make in a small batch. However, it's quick and easy!

INGREDIENTS:

- 2 egg yolks (use pasture raised eggs here, very important)
- 1 tsp. Dijon mustard
- 3 tsp. fresh lemon juice
- ½ cup extra virgin olive oil
- ½ cup coconut oil

INSTRUCTIONS:

1. In a food processor or blender, mix the egg yolks, mustard and half of your lemon juice until smooth.
2. Now, with the blender or food processor on its' lowest setting, begin slowly adding your olive and coconut oils. Be sure not to add too much at once, as this can ruin your end product. Blend nonstop until all oil is eventually added and the mayonnaise has a thick consistency.
3. Lastly, add the rest of your lemon juice and season with salt and pepper to taste. Done!

Egg Salad
Serves: 2

Here is a quick and healthy alternative to your standard egg salad! Eggs are one of the most complete sources of protein available; in other words, they have a complete amino acid profile. This version is made with the same homemade mayonnaise described above, bell pepper and avocado.

INGREDIENTS:

- 4 hardboiled eggs, finely chopped
- 1 tbsp. fresh chives, finely chopped
- ¼ cup homemade mayonnaise
- ¼ cup bell peppers (raw or roasted)
- ¼ tsp. paprika
- salt and pepper to taste

INSTRUCTIONS:

1. Simply mix all ingredients in a bowl aside from the mayonnaise, salt and pepper. Mix together thoroughly.

78

2. Next, mix in the mayo until all is evenly combined.

3. Season to taste with salt and pepper, and place in the fridge for about one hour.

Refreshing Cucumber Salad
Serves: 8

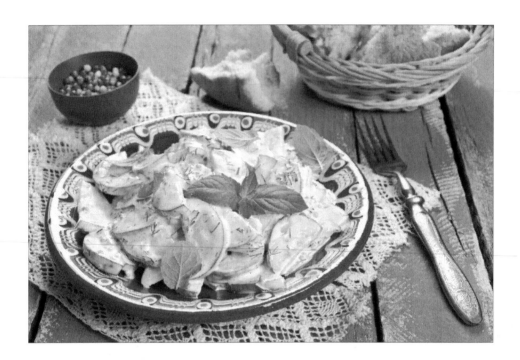

Interestingly enough, while cucumbers have a reputation of not having much nutritional value, they are rich in lignans, which have been connected with cardiovascular health and cancer prevention. This salad is light, but you can always add a protein like hardboiled eggs or chicken, if you want something a bit more filling.

INGREDIENTS:

- 3 cucumbers, thinly sliced
- 1 red onion, thinly sliced
- 3 tbsp. lemon juice
- 3 tbsp. whole fat plain yogurt
- salt and pepper to taste
- 1 tsp. honey
- 1 tsp. chopped cilantro

INSTRUCTIONS:

1. Whisk or thoroughly stir together all ingredients in a bowl except for cucumbers and onion.
2. Once all is thoroughly mixed, add cucumbers and onion, mixing well.
3. That's all! Add protein if desired, and enjoy.

Delicious Crockpot Chicken

Serves: 4-6

A crock-pot is really a miracle invention when it comes to making complex meals incredibly simple. Add the ingredients to your crock-pot (slow-cooker), go to work, and return to an aromatic smelling kitchen and dinner waiting! This great recipe includes the nutrient benefits and sweet taste of yams or sweet potatoes, mixed with chicken and healthy fats from olive oil. Depending on how many people you're feeding, you are likely to have leftovers for the rest of the week.

INGREDIENTS:

- 1 whole chicken
- 3 yams or sweet potatoes (or 5 small)
- salt and pepper to taste
- 2 tbsp. extra virgin olive oil

INSTRUCTIONS:

1. First, wash your sweet potatoes and coat with a bit of your oil, salt and pepper.
2. Wrap them in tin foil and place in your crock pot.
3. Next, top chicken with the rest of your oil, salt and pepper, placing it in the crock pot on top of the sweet potatoes.
4. Allow to cook on low for as few as 4, or up to 7 hours.
5. Once you're ready, simply remove and enjoy! The chicken will have fallen apart and be deliciously tender.

Chicken Salad with Cashews
Serves: 4

A quick yet hearty salad option, this recipe is rich in flavor and simple to prepare. This salad offers the nutrient benefits of the cashew nut (which are actually a seed, contrary to popular belief), that are high in copper, phosphorous, magnesium and zinc. They are also rich in healthy fats, so this salad will keep you satiated.

INGREDIENTS:

- 2 cups cooked chicken, chopped (store-bought or cooked at home prior to meal)
- ½ cup paleo mayo (see above recipe)
- ¼ cup coconut cream or full fat cream (organic, grass-fed if possible)
- 1 red onion, finely chopped
- ¼ cup celery, chopped
- ½ cup roasted cashews, chopped
- ½ cup cilantro, chopped
- juice from 1 fresh lemon
- salt and pepper to taste

INSTRUCTIONS:

1. In a mixing bowl, combine mayo and cream, whisking together. Then, add in onion, celery, cashews, cilantro and lemon juice. Mix everything together thoroughly.
2. Next, add chicken along with salt and pepper, and stir.
3. Serve on top of a green salad (greens of your choice), along with whatever veggies you have laying around the house. I like tomatoes, red bell pepper and avocado. Yum!

Chocolate Cherry Chia Smoothie
Serves: 1

While smoothies are often considered a breakfast food, I enjoy a healthy smoothie as a lunch replacement if I'm really in a rush. This smoothie is satiating and includes chia seeds, which are high in good fats. You also get the antioxidant benefits from cacao, and protein from a high quality protein powder. While I don't suggest a smoothie every day for lunch, it's good to have a few go to recipes on hand in a pinch.

INGREDIENTS:

- 1 cup frozen pitted cherries
- 1½ cup coconut milk (you could also use regular or almond milk)
- 1 tablespoon ground chia seeds
- 1 teaspoon unsweetened cocoa powder OR raw cacao powder
- 1 scoop chocolate protein powder
- 1 tablespoon honey (if you prefer sweeter)

INSTRUCTIONS:

Simply blend all together and enjoy.

Giant Salad
Serves: 1

My go-to lunch choice, particularly when I don't have dinner leftovers, is a giant salad. It is pretty self-explanatory, and can really consist of any vegetables and protein sources you have in the fridge. I have suggested several ideas that I love to throw together, and this can be a super healthy, quick lunch option. If you chop veggies ahead of time to use throughout the week, this process is even easier!

INGREDIENTS:

- 2-3 cups leafy greens (spinach, kale, chard, lettuce, mustard greens, arugula, etc)
- Protein: 2 hardboiled eggs, 4-6 oz chicken, turkey, beef or fish, 1 can wild salmon or tuna, etc.
- Chopped veggies of your choice: bell pepper, cucumber, tomato, carrot, beet, etc.
- ½ avocado, sliced
- 1 tbsp. raw nuts or seeds of your choice (pumpkin, sunflower, walnuts, almonds, etc.)
- olive oil and balsamic vinegar for dressing

INSTRUCTIONS:

Wash all veggies, chop and mix together in a salad bowl and serve!

Quesadilla
Serves: 2

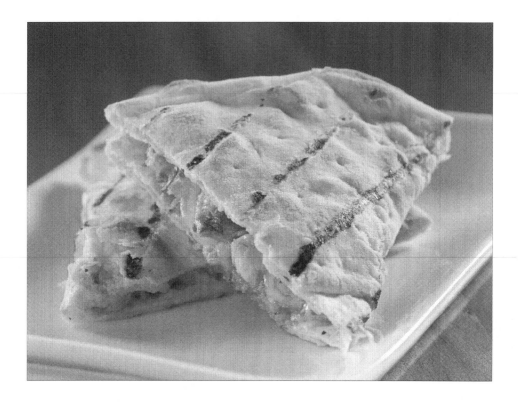

This is another go-to for many people, but there are ways to make this option quite a bit healthier. Instead of using a white flour tortilla, opt for organic corn tortillas, or a whole wheat or sprouted grain gluten-free option. I also like to add beans and veggies to this recipe in order to up the nutrient content.

INGREDIENTS:

- 4-8 corn tortillas (or 4 larger whole wheat or sprouted grain tortillas)
- shredded cheese of your choice (enough to create a thin later on your tortilla)
- 1 avocado, sliced
- ½ can black beans, rinsed and drained
- 2 handfuls spinach, washed and chopped
- 1 tbsp. extra virgin olive oil

INSTRUCTIONS:

1. Heat olive oil in a sauté pan on medium heat.
2. Once hot, place one tortilla in the pan, and top with cheese, black beans and spinach. Cover with second tortilla.
3. Press down with a spatula, allowing to cook for about 2-3 minutes. Now, flip and cook on the other side for another 2 minutes.
4. Remove from heat, and repeat process with second quesadilla (if feeding 2 people).
5. Top with sliced avocado and enjoy!

The Lunchbox
Serves: 1

Remember when you were a kid and your mom packed your lunchbox? That tradition doesn't need to stop after childhood! Your lunchbox can include leftovers from last night's dinner, chopped fruit and vegetables, nuts and seeds, a healthy sandwich and more. I try to add raw sauerkraut as a side to my lunchbox, as it provides healthy probiotics, which are essential to digestive health. Here are some of my favorite lunchbox additions.

INGREDIENTS:

- Homemade trail mix: small handful of nuts (almonds, walnuts, etc), dried cranberries, and unsweetened coconut flakes
- 1 pre-cooked and chopped organic sausage (I like applegate organics brand)
- Chopped carrots, broccoli, and tomato
- ½ cup raw sauerkraut

INSTRUCTIONS:

Arrange in your lunchbox and pack!

Before you go, I'd like to remind you that there is a free, complimentary eBook waiting for you. Download it today to treat yourself to healthy, <u>gluten-free desserts and snacks</u> so that you never feel deprived again!

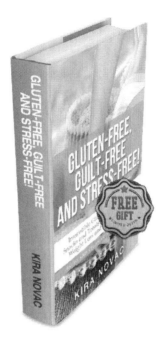

Download link

http://bit.ly/gluten-free-desserts-book

Conclusion

This concludes our anti-inflammatory lunch recipe book, and I hope you take from it some new, fun and exciting ideas for how to easily incorporate anti-inflammatory foods into your daily diet. Remember, changing your diet does not need take place overnight, it can be a slower process that creates sustainable, lifelong change. The wonderful thing about eating anti-inflammatory foods is that there is simply *so* much to choose from! Whether you are eating a paleo, vegetarian, vegan or other type of diet, there are plenty of nutrient dense, healthy and anti-inflammatory choices to make. And, recipes can range from intricate and complicated to quick and simple, depending on your preferences, lifestyle and obligations.

As always, have fun, experiment, and don't be afraid to try new things. Your body will reap the benefits in the short and long term.

Please rank this book on Amazon and post a short review to let me know your favorite recipes. I'd be extremely happy to hear from you!

I am here to help you.

Remember, the beauty of incorporating anti-inflammatory foods into your daily diet is that you are making not only healthy, but sustainable changes. In reducing systemic inflammation in the body, you are working to prevent potential diseases such as cancer, diabetes, arthritis and many more. You are also providing your children with the crucial nutrient base they need to grow into happy, healthy adults.

As with any dietary changes, this is a process. Be kind to yourself, and know you are taking important steps on the road to health and wellness.

To your success,

Kira

To post an honest review

One more thing... If you have received any value from this book, can you please rank it and post a short review? It only takes a few seconds really and it would really make my day. It's you I am writing for and your opinion is always much appreciated. In order to do so;

1. Log into your account
2. Search for my book on Amazon or check your orders / or go to my author page at:

http://amazon.com/author/kira-novac

3. Click on a book you have read, then click on "reviews" and "create your review".

Please let me know your favorite motivational tip you learned from this book.

If you happen to have any questions or doubts about this book, please e-mail me at:

kira.novac@kiraglutenfreerecipes.com

I would love to hear from you!

Recommended Reading

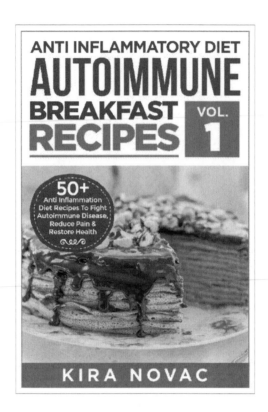

Book Link:

http://bit.ly/af-breakfast-recipes

Recommended Reading

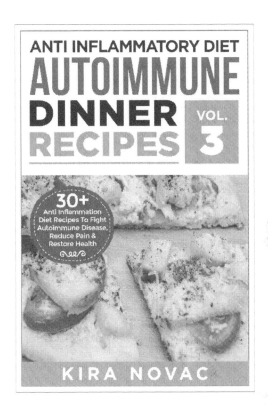

Book Link:

http://bit.ly/af-dinner-recipes

FOR MORE HEALTH BOOKS (KINDLE & PAPERBACK) BY KIRA NOVAC PLEASE VISIT:

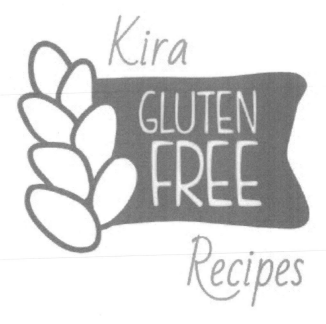

www.kiraglutenfreerecipes.com/books

Thank you for taking an interest in my work,

Kira and Holistic Wellness Books

HOLISTIC WELLNESS & HEALTH BOOKS

If you are interested in health, wellness, spirituality and personal development, visit our page and be the first one to know about free and 0.99 eBooks:

www.HolisticWellnessBooks.com

Made in the USA
Lexington, KY
10 July 2018